The Future of Medicine in Clinical Innovations and Trends

Elena Einstein

Title: The Future of Medicine in Germany Innovations and Trends

Author's: Elena Einstein.

This book was printed and published by [Publisher's: Elena Einstein] in [2023]

ISBN:

TABLE OF CONTENTS

Chapter 8: Future Challenges and Opportunities

60

Aging Population and Geriatric Healthcare

Mental Health and Psychiatric Care

Integrating Traditional and Modern Medicine

Global Collaboration and Medical Diplomacy

Chapter 9: Conclusion

68

Summary of Findings

Implications for the Future of Medicine in Germany

Recommendations for Policy and Practice

Chapter 1: Introduction

Background and Significance

Germany has long been recognized as a global leader in the field of medicine, with a rich history of scientific breakthroughs and high-quality healthcare. The Future of Medicine in Germany: Innovations and Trends explores the current landscape of the medical scope in Germany and the significant advancements that are shaping the future of healthcare in the country.

The German healthcare system is renowned for its excellence and efficiency, providing comprehensive medical care to its citizens. With a strong emphasis on research and innovation, Germany has consistently been at the forefront of medical advancements, pioneering groundbreaking treatments and technologies. This book delves into the background and significance of these advancements, shedding light on the key developments that have put Germany at the forefront of the global medical community.

One of the key areas of focus is the rise of digital health technologies in Germany. The integration of digital tools and solutions into healthcare has transformed the way medical professionals deliver care and patients access it. From telemedicine and remote monitoring to electronic health records and virtual reality applications, Germany has embraced digital health with open arms. This subchapter explores the background and significance of these digital innovations, discussing how they are revolutionizing the medical scope in Germany and improving patient outcomes.

Another crucial aspect covered in this subchapter is the significance of medical research and its impact on the future of medicine in Germany.

Germany boasts world-class research institutions and universities that are dedicated to advancing medical knowledge and finding breakthrough treatments for various diseases. The subchapter sheds light on the importance of medical research, discussing the major research initiatives and collaborations that are driving innovation in the country.

Furthermore, the subchapter also presents an overview of the German healthcare system, highlighting its unique characteristics and strengths. It delves into the structure of the system, including the role of health insurance and the various healthcare providers. By understanding the background and significance of the German healthcare system, readers gain a deeper appreciation of how medical advancements and trends are shaping the future of healthcare in Germany.

In conclusion, the subchapter on Background and Significance offers an insightful exploration of the medical scope in Germany. It provides readers with a comprehensive understanding of the historical context, significance of medical research, digital health advancements, and the unique healthcare system in Germany. Whether you are a medical professional, a researcher, or simply interested in the future of medicine, this subchapter offers valuable insights into the innovations and trends that are shaping the future of healthcare in Germany.

Purpose and Objectives

The Purpose and Objectives of this subchapter are to provide a comprehensive understanding of the medical scope in Germany, addressing the audience of all individuals interested in the future of medicine and healthcare innovations in the country.

Germany has long been recognized as a global leader in medical research, innovation, and patient care. This subchapter aims to shed light on the current state of the German healthcare system and its future direction.

The primary objective is to explore the various innovations and trends that are shaping the future of medicine in Germany. From advancements in technology to changes in healthcare policies, this subchapter will delve into the factors that are driving transformation in the medical field.

Another objective of this subchapter is to highlight the significant role played by medical professionals, researchers, and scientists in Germany. It will provide insights into the cutting-edge research being conducted in the country, as well as the collaboration between academia, industry, and healthcare providers.

Furthermore, the subchapter will delve into the challenges faced by the German healthcare system. It will explore issues such as rising healthcare costs, an aging population, and the need for sustainable healthcare solutions. It aims to provide a comprehensive overview of the obstacles that need to be overcome to ensure a robust and efficient healthcare system for the future.

The subchapter will also examine the role of digitalization in the German healthcare system. With the advent of technologies such as telemedicine, electronic health records, and artificial intelligence, the way healthcare is delivered and managed is rapidly evolving. This section will explore the potential benefits of digitalization and the challenges that come with it.

Moreover, the subchapter will discuss the importance of international collaboration in medical research and innovation. Germany has been at the forefront of international cooperation, and this section will shed light on the partnerships and initiatives that are driving global advancements in medicine.

In conclusion, this subchapter aims to provide a comprehensive overview of the purpose and objectives of the book "The Future of Medicine in Germany: Innovations and Trends." It will analyze the current state of the medical scope in Germany, explore the future direction of healthcare, and highlight the challenges and opportunities that lie ahead. Whether you are a medical professional, researcher, policymaker, or simply someone interested in the future of medicine, this subchapter will provide valuable insights into the advancements and trends shaping the German healthcare system.

Scope and Limitations

In the ever-evolving field of medicine, it is essential to understand the scope and limitations of medical practice in Germany. As advancements in technology and research pave the way for new innovations and trends, it becomes crucial for healthcare professionals, policymakers, and patients to be aware of the possibilities and constraints within the German medical system.

The scope of medical practice in Germany encompasses a wide range of specialties and sub-specialties. With a strong emphasis on evidence-based medicine, German physicians are highly trained and skilled in providing quality healthcare services. From general practitioners to specialists in fields such as cardiology, oncology, neurology, and many others, the German medical system offers a comprehensive approach to patient care.

One of the key strengths of the German medical scope is its emphasis on research and innovation. Germany is known for its world-class academic institutions, cutting-edge medical research, and a robust pharmaceutical industry. This enables physicians to stay at the forefront of medical advancements and offer state-of-the-art treatments to patients.

However, it is important to note that the scope of medical practice in Germany is not without limitations. Despite the country's well-established healthcare system, there are challenges that need to be addressed. One such limitation is the increasing demand for healthcare services due to an aging population and the rise of chronic diseases. This puts pressure on the healthcare system, leading to longer waiting times for specialized treatments and surgeries.

Another limitation is the regional disparity in healthcare access. While urban areas boast excellent medical facilities and resources, rural regions struggle with limited access to healthcare services. This discrepancy poses challenges in providing equitable healthcare to all citizens across Germany.

Furthermore, the German medical system is subject to financial constraints. As healthcare costs continue to rise, funding and reimbursement models need to be carefully managed to ensure sustainable and affordable healthcare for the population. Balancing the quality and accessibility of medical services while keeping healthcare costs in check is an ongoing challenge for policymakers and healthcare professionals.

In conclusion, understanding the scope and limitations of the medical practice in Germany is crucial for all stakeholders in the healthcare ecosystem. The German medical system offers a wide range of specialties and is known for its research and innovation. However, challenges such as increasing demand, regional disparities, and financial constraints need to be addressed to ensure the future of medicine in Germany is sustainable and accessible to all. By being aware of these limitations, we can work towards overcoming them and fostering a healthcare system that meets the needs of patients and providers alike.

Chapter 2: Overview of the Medical Landscape in Germany

Historical Development of Medicine in Germany

Germany has a rich and storied history when it comes to the development of medicine. From ancient times to the modern era, this nation has made significant contributions to the field of healthcare and continues to be a leader in medical advancement. Understanding the historical development of medicine in Germany is crucial for anyone interested in the medical scope in Germany.

Ancient Germany was home to various tribes and civilizations that practiced traditional healing methods. These practices involved the use of herbal remedies, spiritual rituals, and primitive surgical techniques. However, it was during the Medieval period that Germany began to emerge as a center for medical education and innovation.

The establishment of universities across Germany, such as the University of Padua and the University of Leipzig, played a pivotal role in the development of medicine. These institutions became renowned for their medical programs and attracted scholars from all over Europe. It was during this time that the foundations of modern medicine were laid, with advancements in anatomy, physiology, and pharmacology.

In the 19th century, Germany witnessed significant breakthroughs in medical research and practice. The development of the microscope allowed scientists to study cells and microorganisms, leading to groundbreaking discoveries in the field of microbiology. Prominent German physicians, such as Robert Koch and Rudolf Virchow, made remarkable contributions to the understanding and treatment of infectious diseases.

Furthermore, the concept of evidence-based medicine was introduced in Germany during this period. The idea that medical decisions should be based on scientific evidence and clinical expertise revolutionized the healthcare industry and became a cornerstone of modern medical practice.

In the 20th century, Germany faced challenging times with the rise of the Nazi regime. The medical community was forced to confront the horrors of unethical medical experimentation and the persecution of Jewish physicians. However, in the aftermath of World War II, Germany embarked on a journey of rebuilding and reforming its healthcare system.

Today, Germany is recognized as a global leader in medical innovation and research. The country boasts world-class medical facilities, cutting-edge technology, and a strong commitment to patient care. German scientists and physicians continue to make groundbreaking discoveries in various fields, including genetics, immunology, and oncology.

The historical development of medicine in Germany showcases the nation's resilience and determination to advance healthcare for the betterment of society. As the future of medicine unfolds, Germany remains at the forefront of medical innovation, providing hope for a healthier tomorrow.

In conclusion, the historical development of medicine in Germany is a fascinating journey that has shaped the medical scope in the country. From ancient healing traditions to modern advancements, Germany has been at the forefront of medical innovation. By understanding this history, individuals can gain a deeper appreciation for the contributions of Germany to the field of medicine and the potential for future innovations and trends.

Current Healthcare System in Germany

Germany is renowned for its high-quality healthcare system, which is often considered one of the best in the world. This subchapter aims to provide an overview of the current healthcare system in Germany, with a focus on the medical scope in the country. Whether you are a medical professional, a patient, or simply interested in healthcare, this information will give you valuable insights into how healthcare is organized and delivered in Germany.

The German healthcare system operates under a dual system, combining statutory health insurance (SHI) and private health insurance (PHI). Approximately 90% of the population is covered by SHI, while the remaining 10% opt for PHI. SHI is mandatory for individuals with a gross income below a certain threshold, while PHI is primarily chosen by high-income earners and the self-employed.

One of the key features of the German healthcare system is its emphasis on universal coverage, ensuring that everyone has access to healthcare services. Medical care in Germany is comprehensive, encompassing preventive care, outpatient care, inpatient care, and rehabilitation services. Patients have the freedom to choose their healthcare providers, whether it be general practitioners, specialists, or hospitals.

Germany boasts a highly specialized and well-trained medical workforce. Medical education and training in Germany are rigorous, with medical professionals required to undergo extensive studies and practical training. This emphasis on education and specialization contributes to the high standard of medical care provided in the country.

In terms of medical innovations and trends, Germany is at the forefront of research and development. The country has a robust pharmaceutical and biotechnology industry, fostering continuous advancements in medical treatments and technologies. From cutting-edge surgical procedures to innovative medical devices, Germany's healthcare system consistently integrates new approaches to improve patient outcomes and quality of care.

Moreover, Germany places great importance on digital health and telemedicine. The country has been actively investing in digital infrastructure and promoting the use of electronic health records, teleconsultations, and remote monitoring. These digital solutions not only enhance efficiency in healthcare delivery but also facilitate better access to healthcare, particularly in rural areas.

In conclusion, the current healthcare system in Germany encompasses universal coverage, a well-trained medical workforce, and a strong focus on medical innovations and trends. This subchapter aimed to provide an overview of the medical scope in Germany, highlighting the comprehensive care, freedom of choice, and emphasis on education and specialization. Whether you are a medical professional or a patient, understanding the German healthcare system is essential for navigating the intricacies of healthcare delivery in the country.

Key Players in the Medical Field

In the rapidly evolving landscape of the medical field, Germany has emerged as a global leader in healthcare innovation and technology. This subchapter aims to introduce the key players who are shaping the future of medicine in Germany. From research institutions to pharmaceutical companies, these influential organizations are driving advancements and trends that impact the medical scope in Germany.

Research Institutions:

Germany boasts a robust network of research institutions dedicated to medical advancements. One such institution is the Max Planck Society, renowned for its groundbreaking research in various scientific disciplines, including medicine. The Helmholtz Association is another key player in medical research, focusing on topics such as personalized medicine and biomedical engineering. These institutions not only contribute to cutting-edge medical discoveries but also foster collaborations with universities and industry partners.

Pharmaceutical Companies:

The pharmaceutical industry plays a vital role in the medical field, and Germany is home to several prominent companies. Bayer, a global pharmaceutical giant, has a strong presence in Germany, specializing in areas such as cardiology, oncology, and women's health. Merck, another major player, is known for its innovative medicines and vaccines, with a focus on therapeutic areas like neurology, oncology, and immunology. These companies invest heavily in research and development, ensuring that new treatments and therapies reach patients.

Medical Technology:

Germany is renowned for its expertise and innovation in medical technology. Siemens Healthineers, a global leader in medical imaging, laboratory diagnostics, and healthcare IT, is a prominent player in this field. Their cutting-edge solutions enable precise diagnostics and efficient healthcare delivery. Additionally, companies like B. Braun and Fresenius Medical Care are known for their contributions to medical devices and renal therapies, respectively. These companies continuously strive to enhance patient care and improve treatment outcomes.

Start-ups and Innovators:

The German medical field also thrives on the contributions of start-ups and innovators. Numerous young companies are disrupting traditional healthcare models with digital health solutions, telemedicine platforms, and AI-driven diagnostics. For instance, Ada Health has developed an AI-powered symptom assessment tool, enabling users to receive personalized health advice. Another notable start-up, TeleClinic, offers remote consultations with certified physicians, revolutionizing access to healthcare services.

These key players in the medical field are at the forefront of driving innovations and trends in Germany. They collaborate with researchers, healthcare professionals, and regulatory bodies to develop new treatments, improve patient care, and shape the future of medicine. By harnessing the potential of technology, research, and pharmaceutical expertise, Germany continues to lead the way in medical innovation, making significant contributions to the medical scope not only in Germany but also globally.

Challenges and Opportunities

Germany has long been recognized as a global leader in the field of medicine, with a rich history of groundbreaking discoveries and innovations. However, like any other country, it also faces its fair share of challenges in the ever-evolving healthcare landscape. This subchapter explores the challenges and opportunities that lie ahead for the future of medicine in Germany, shedding light on the path forward for both the medical community and the general public.

One of the major challenges faced by the medical scope in Germany is the increasing burden of an aging population. As life expectancy continues to rise, the demand for healthcare services, particularly in geriatric care, is expected to skyrocket. This poses challenges for healthcare professionals who need to ensure that they have the necessary resources and infrastructure to cater to the needs of this growing demographic. Innovative approaches, such as telemedicine and home healthcare, are being explored to address these challenges and provide efficient and accessible care to the elderly.

Another challenge that Germany faces is the rising cost of healthcare. With advancements in medical technology, the cost of treatments and medications has surged, putting pressure on the healthcare system. This necessitates a comprehensive review of the healthcare financing model and the exploration of alternative funding mechanisms to ensure sustainable and affordable healthcare for all.

However, amidst these challenges, Germany also presents numerous opportunities for the future of medicine. The country boasts a robust research and development sector, with top-notch universities and research institutions that foster innovation and scientific discovery. This provides a fertile ground for the development of cutting-edge therapies and treatments that can revolutionize healthcare in Germany and beyond.

Moreover, Germany has a strong tradition of collaboration between academia, industry, and the government. This collaborative approach can pave the way for interdisciplinary research and foster the translation of scientific discoveries into clinical practice. Partnerships between pharmaceutical companies, medical device manufacturers, and healthcare providers can help accelerate the development and adoption of innovative medical technologies, ultimately improving patient outcomes.

The future of medicine in Germany holds immense potential. By addressing the challenges and capitalizing on the opportunities, the country can continue to be at the forefront of medical advancements and provide high-quality healthcare to its citizens. This subchapter aims to inspire the medical community and the wider public to embrace the challenges and seize the opportunities that lie ahead, fostering a culture of innovation and excellence in healthcare delivery.

Chapter 3: Innovations in Medical Research and Technology

Advancements in Biotechnology

Biotechnology has been at the forefront of medical innovation, revolutionizing the way we diagnose, treat, and prevent diseases. In Germany, the field of biotechnology has witnessed significant advancements, shaping the future of medicine in the country. This subchapter explores the latest trends and innovations in biotechnology and their impact on the medical scope in Germany.

One of the most remarkable advancements in biotechnology is the development of personalized medicine. Through the analysis of an individual's genetic makeup, scientists can now tailor treatments to specific patients, ensuring greater efficacy and fewer side effects. This personalized approach has transformed the way diseases such as cancer, diabetes, and rare genetic disorders are managed in Germany, leading to improved patient outcomes.

Another breakthrough in biotechnology is the development of gene editing techniques like CRISPR-Cas9. This revolutionary technology allows scientists to modify genes with unprecedented precision, opening new avenues for treating genetic diseases. Germany has been at the forefront of gene editing research, with numerous institutions and companies actively exploring its potential applications in medicine.

Biotechnology has also played a pivotal role in the development of advanced diagnostics. Germany has witnessed a surge in the development of innovative diagnostic tools that can detect diseases at an early stage, leading to timely interventions and improved prognosis. From advanced imaging techniques to rapid diagnostic tests, biotechnology has empowered healthcare professionals in Germany with powerful tools to accurately diagnose and monitor diseases.

Furthermore, biotechnology has significantly contributed to the development of novel therapeutics. Germany has witnessed the rise of biopharmaceutical companies that utilize biotechnological processes to produce highly effective drugs. These biologics, derived from living organisms, have revolutionized the treatment of diseases such as cancer, autoimmune disorders, and infectious diseases, offering new hope to patients across the country.

In conclusion, advancements in biotechnology have transformed the medical scope in Germany. Personalized medicine, gene editing, advanced diagnostics, and novel therapeutics are just a few examples of the remarkable progress made in this field. As Germany continues to embrace and invest in biotechnology, it is poised to remain a leader in medical innovation, offering improved healthcare outcomes for all.

Breakthroughs in Pharmaceutical Research

In the fast-paced world of medicine, pharmaceutical research plays a critical role in advancing healthcare and improving patient outcomes. Germany, known for its strong medical infrastructure and commitment to innovation, has been at the forefront of groundbreaking discoveries in the field. This subchapter explores some of the most significant breakthroughs in pharmaceutical research that have emerged from Germany, shedding light on the exciting future of medicine in the country.

One notable breakthrough in pharmaceutical research is the development of targeted therapies. Scientists in Germany have made remarkable strides in identifying specific molecular targets within the body that contribute to the development and progression of diseases such as cancer. By designing drugs that specifically target these molecular markers, researchers have been able to create more effective and personalized treatment options. These targeted therapies not only enhance patient outcomes but also reduce the side effects associated with traditional treatments.

Another breakthrough that has revolutionized medicine in Germany is the advent of precision medicine. By integrating genetic information with clinical data, researchers are able to predict an individual's response to certain medications, allowing for tailored treatment plans. This approach has proved particularly effective in areas such as oncology, where treatment decisions can be optimized based on a patient's genetic profile. Precision medicine has the potential to significantly improve patient care, minimize adverse reactions, and streamline healthcare delivery.

Furthermore, Germany is at the forefront of research into novel drug delivery systems. Scientists have been exploring innovative methods to improve drug efficacy and reduce toxicity. Nanotechnology, for instance, has shown promise in delivering drugs directly to diseased cells, minimizing damage to healthy tissue. This approach has the potential to revolutionize drug delivery, enabling more targeted and efficient treatments.

Moreover, Germany has made significant contributions to the development of immunotherapy, a groundbreaking approach that harnesses the body's immune system to fight diseases. From the development of immune checkpoint inhibitors to personalized cancer vaccines, German researchers have spearheaded advancements in this field, offering new hope to patients with previously untreatable conditions.

As Germany continues to foster a collaborative environment for pharmaceutical research, the future of medicine in the country looks promising. Through ongoing innovation and investment in cutting-edge technologies, Germany is poised to remain a global leader in medical research and healthcare delivery. The breakthroughs discussed in this subchapter represent just a glimpse into the transformative potential of pharmaceutical research in Germany, and the impact it will have on the medical scope in the country and beyond.

In conclusion, the remarkable breakthroughs in pharmaceutical research emerging from Germany are transforming the landscape of medicine. From targeted therapies to precision medicine, novel drug delivery systems to immunotherapy, these advancements have the potential to revolutionize patient care and improve health outcomes.

As the future unfolds, Germany's commitment to innovation and collaboration ensures that the country will continue to be at the forefront of pharmaceutical research, driving the medical scope in Germany to new heights.

Cutting-Edge Medical Devices and Equipment

In recent years, Germany has emerged as a global leader in the field of medical technology, boasting a remarkable array of cutting-edge medical devices and equipment. These innovations have revolutionized the healthcare industry and have paved the way for unprecedented advancements in patient care and treatment. This subchapter will delve into the exciting world of medical technology in Germany and explore the innovations and trends that are shaping the future of medicine in the country.

Germany's commitment to research and development has set the stage for groundbreaking medical inventions. From state-of-the-art imaging devices to robotic surgical systems, German engineers and scientists have been at the forefront of medical device innovation, constantly pushing the boundaries of what is possible. These cutting-edge devices not only enhance accuracy and precision in diagnosis and treatment but also improve patient outcomes and quality of life.

One of the notable advancements in medical technology is the development of minimally invasive surgical techniques. German medical device companies have pioneered the creation of robotic surgical systems that allow surgeons to perform complex procedures with greater precision and minimal invasiveness. These systems enable surgeons to make smaller incisions, leading to reduced scarring, faster recovery times, and less post-operative pain for patients.

Another area of innovation lies in diagnostic imaging. German manufacturers have introduced advanced imaging technologies such as magnetic resonance imaging (MRI) machines, computed tomography (CT) scanners, and ultrasound devices that provide detailed and accurate images of the human body. These devices have revolutionized the field of medical diagnostics, allowing for early detection of diseases and conditions, leading to more effective and timely treatments.

Moreover, Germany has been at the forefront of developing wearable medical devices and digital health solutions. These devices, such as smartwatches, fitness trackers, and remote patient monitoring systems, have the potential to transform healthcare by enabling continuous monitoring of vital signs, tracking fitness levels, and providing real-time health data to both patients and healthcare providers. This integration of technology with healthcare has the potential to improve the management of chronic diseases and facilitate remote patient care.

In conclusion, Germany's medical technology industry is a hotbed of innovation, constantly pushing the boundaries of what is possible in patient care and treatment. From robotic surgical systems to advanced diagnostic imaging devices and wearable health technologies, German medical device manufacturers are at the forefront of revolutionizing healthcare. The future of medicine in Germany looks bright, with cutting-edge medical devices and equipment playing a pivotal role in improving patient outcomes and pushing the boundaries of medical science. Whether you are a healthcare professional, patient, or simply interested in medical advancements, exploring the world of medical technology in Germany is a journey worth taking.

Digitalization and Artificial Intelligence in Healthcare

In recent years, the healthcare industry has witnessed an exponential growth in digitalization and the integration of artificial intelligence (AI) technologies. This subchapter aims to explore the impact of these advancements on the medical scope in Germany.

Germany, known for its world-class healthcare system, has embraced digitalization and AI to enhance patient care, improve efficiency, and drive innovation. The integration of digital technologies in healthcare has resulted in numerous benefits, making medical services more accessible and personalized.

One of the key advantages of digitalization is the ability to collect and analyze vast amounts of patient data. This data, when combined with AI algorithms, can provide valuable insights for diagnosis, treatment, and prevention. AI-powered systems are capable of identifying patterns and anomalies in medical records, enabling early detection of diseases and improving accuracy in diagnosis. This not only saves lives but also reduces healthcare costs by preventing unnecessary treatments.

Moreover, digitalization has revolutionized patient-doctor interactions. Telemedicine, for instance, has emerged as a convenient and efficient way to provide medical consultations remotely. Patients can now communicate with healthcare professionals via video calls, eliminating the need for physical visits. This is particularly beneficial for rural areas, where access to medical facilities may be limited. The integration of AI in telemedicine further enhances the experience by providing automated symptom analysis and suggestions for further actions.

In addition to improving patient care, digitalization and AI have also transformed healthcare management. Electronic health records (EHRs) have replaced traditional paper-based systems, ensuring seamless and secure access to patient information for healthcare providers. This streamlines processes, reduces administrative burdens, and enables better coordination among medical professionals. AI-powered chatbots have also been introduced to handle routine inquiries, freeing up human resources to focus on more complex tasks.

While digitalization and AI bring remarkable advancements, it is crucial to address the challenges they present. Privacy concerns, data security, and ethical considerations are some of the key issues that need to be carefully managed. Furthermore, it is essential to ensure that these technologies are accessible to all, bridging the digital divide and preventing inequality in healthcare access.

In conclusion, the digitalization and integration of AI in healthcare have revolutionized the medical scope in Germany. These advancements have improved patient care, enhanced efficiency, and paved the way for personalized medicine. As the future unfolds, it is vital to continue exploring the potential of digitalization and AI, while addressing the associated challenges, to ensure a sustainable and inclusive healthcare system for all in Germany.

Chapter 4: Promising Trends in Medical Education and Training

Medical Schools and Universities in Germany

Germany is renowned for its exceptional education system, and its medical schools and universities are no exception. With a rich history in medical research and innovation, Germany continues to attract students from all over the world who are aspiring to pursue a career in the field of medicine. In this subchapter, we will explore the medical scope in Germany and the various academic institutions that offer medical education.

Germany is home to numerous prestigious medical schools and universities that provide comprehensive medical programs and cutting-edge research opportunities. These institutions offer a wide range of courses, including undergraduate and postgraduate programs, as well as specialized medical training for those pursuing specialization in specific fields. The curriculum is designed to provide students with a strong foundation in medical knowledge, clinical skills, and research methodologies.

One of the most renowned medical schools in Germany is the Charité - Universitätsmedizin Berlin, which is not only a leading institution in the country but also enjoys international recognition. It combines the expertise of four different medical faculties and offers a diverse range of medical programs. Another prominent institution is the University of Heidelberg, known for its strong emphasis on research and collaboration with renowned medical institutions.

In addition to these, Germany boasts several other prestigious medical schools and universities, such as the Ludwig Maximilian University of

Munich, the University of Freiburg, and the University of Tübingen. These institutions are known for their state-of-the-art facilities, experienced faculty members, and collaborative research opportunities.

Studying medicine in Germany not only provides students with a high-quality education but also opens up numerous career opportunities. Upon graduation, medical students have the option to pursue further specialization or enter the workforce directly. The German healthcare system is highly advanced, ensuring that medical professionals are in high demand. Moreover, Germany's progressive healthcare policies and emphasis on research and innovation make it an attractive destination for medical professionals.

In conclusion, Germany's medical schools and universities offer excellent opportunities for students aspiring to pursue a career in medicine. With a robust curriculum, state-of-the-art facilities, and a rich research culture, these institutions provide students with a solid foundation to excel in their medical careers. Whether it is clinical practice, research, or specialization, Germany offers a wide range of options for medical professionals.

Curriculum and Training Programs

In the rapidly evolving field of medicine, it is crucial for healthcare professionals to stay up-to-date with the latest innovations and trends. Germany, known for its exceptional healthcare system, places a strong emphasis on the quality of education and training provided to aspiring medical professionals. This subchapter explores the curriculum and training programs in the medical scope in Germany, highlighting the advancements and opportunities available in this field.

Germany's medical curriculum is designed to provide students with a comprehensive understanding of the human body, diseases, and medical treatments. The curriculum is divided into preclinical and clinical phases, ensuring a gradual transition from theoretical knowledge to practical experience. During the preclinical phase, students acquire a solid foundation in basic sciences, including anatomy, physiology, biochemistry, and microbiology. This phase lays the groundwork for the subsequent clinical phase, where students gain hands-on experience through rotations in various medical specialties.

One of the unique aspects of medical education in Germany is the integration of practical training from an early stage. Students have the opportunity to interact with patients in teaching hospitals, enabling them to apply their theoretical knowledge in real-life scenarios. This exposure to clinical settings enhances their clinical skills and fosters a patient-centered approach to healthcare.

Furthermore, Germany offers a wide range of specialized training programs for medical professionals seeking to further enhance their expertise. These programs cater to various medical disciplines, such as cardiology, radiology, orthopedics, and neurology, among others. Through these training programs, medical professionals can deepen their knowledge and acquire advanced skills in their respective fields, ensuring that they remain at the forefront of medical advancements.

To ensure the continuous professional development of medical practitioners, Germany also promotes continuing medical education (CME) programs. These programs provide healthcare professionals with opportunities to attend seminars, workshops, and conferences, where they can learn about the latest innovations, research, and advancements in their areas of interest.

In conclusion, Germany's curriculum and training programs in the medical scope are designed to equip aspiring medical professionals with the necessary knowledge and skills to excel in their careers. The integration of theoretical and practical training, along with specialized training programs and CME opportunities, ensures that healthcare professionals in Germany are well-prepared to meet the challenges of the ever-evolving field of medicine. By investing in quality education and training, Germany continues to drive innovation and contribute to the future of medicine both within its borders and globally.

Interdisciplinary Approaches in Medical Education

In the rapidly evolving field of medicine, interdisciplinary approaches have become increasingly important. As the world becomes more interconnected, healthcare professionals must be equipped with the knowledge and skills to collaborate effectively across various disciplines. This subchapter explores the significance of interdisciplinary approaches in medical education, specifically focusing on the medical scope in Germany.

Germany has long been recognized as a global leader in medical research and innovation. With renowned universities and cutting-edge healthcare facilities, the country offers a fertile ground for interdisciplinary collaboration. Medical education in Germany has embraced this trend, aiming to produce well-rounded professionals who can address complex healthcare challenges through collaboration and innovation.

Interdisciplinary approaches in medical education promote a holistic understanding of healthcare. By integrating knowledge from different fields, such as medicine, psychology, sociology, and engineering, medical students gain a comprehensive perspective that goes beyond a narrow focus on individual diseases. This approach enables them to consider the broader social, cultural, and environmental factors that influence health outcomes, ultimately leading to more effective and patient-centered care.

One example of interdisciplinary education in Germany is the integration of technology and medicine. Rapid advancements in digital health, telemedicine, and artificial intelligence have transformed the healthcare landscape. Medical students are now exposed to these technologies during their training, learning how to leverage them to improve patient care. By collaborating with experts in computer science and engineering, they develop a deeper understanding of these technologies and their potential applications in healthcare.

Another interdisciplinary approach gaining traction in Germany is the integration of social sciences into medical education. Recognizing that health is influenced by social determinants and cultural factors, medical schools are incorporating courses on sociology, anthropology, and ethics. This enables future doctors to better comprehend the social context of their patients' lives and tailor treatment plans accordingly. By understanding the impact of social and cultural factors on health, medical professionals can deliver more equitable and culturally sensitive care.

In conclusion, interdisciplinary approaches in medical education have become essential in the medical scope in Germany. By embracing collaboration across various disciplines, medical schools are preparing future healthcare professionals to address the complex challenges of the 21st century. These approaches promote a holistic understanding of health and enable professionals to provide patient-centered and culturally sensitive care. As Germany continues to lead in medical innovation, interdisciplinary education will play a crucial role in shaping the future of medicine in the country.

Addressing the Physician Shortage

Germany, like many other countries, is facing a significant physician shortage that poses a considerable challenge to its healthcare system. This subchapter explores the various strategies and initiatives that have been implemented to address this pressing issue and ensure the future of the medical scope in Germany.

One of the main factors contributing to the physician shortage is the aging population. As the German population continues to age, the demand for healthcare services increases, placing a strain on the existing workforce. To combat this, efforts have been made to attract more medical students and encourage them to pursue careers in primary care and underserved areas. Scholarships, grants, and financial incentives have been introduced to alleviate the financial burden associated with medical education and encourage students to specialize in fields that are experiencing a shortage.

Another approach to address the physician shortage is the expansion of medical training programs and the promotion of interdisciplinary collaboration. Germany has been working on increasing the number of medical schools and training facilities, allowing for a larger intake of students. Additionally, efforts are being made to foster collaboration between different healthcare professionals, such as nurses, pharmacists, and physicians, to provide comprehensive and efficient care.

Furthermore, the use of technology and advancements in telemedicine have played a crucial role in addressing the physician shortage. Telemedicine allows for remote consultations, diagnosis, and treatment, reducing the need for in-person visits and providing more accessible healthcare services, particularly in rural and underserved areas. This approach has proven to be beneficial, not only in increasing access to care but also in improving patient outcomes.

To ensure the sustainability of the healthcare system and address the physician shortage in the long term, it is essential to foster a supportive and attractive working environment for physicians. This includes addressing concerns such as high workload, burnout, and bureaucratic hurdles. Implementing policies that promote work-life balance, flexible scheduling, and career advancement opportunities can help attract and retain healthcare professionals.

In conclusion, the physician shortage in Germany is a complex issue that requires multifaceted solutions. By investing in medical education, promoting interdisciplinary collaboration, embracing technology, and creating an attractive working environment, Germany can address this challenge and ensure the future of the medical scope in the country. These efforts will not only benefit the healthcare system but also improve the overall well-being of the population and maintain Germany's position as a leader in medical innovation and trends.

Chapter 5: Revolutionizing Patient Care and Treatment

Personalized Medicine and Genomic Research

In recent years, the field of medicine has witnessed a groundbreaking revolution known as personalized medicine, driven by advancements in genomic research. This subchapter aims to provide an overview of personalized medicine and its implications for the medical scope in Germany.

Personalized medicine is an innovative approach that tailors medical treatment to an individual's unique genetic makeup. It recognizes that each person's genetic code is distinct and can influence their response to medications, susceptibility to diseases, and overall health. By analyzing an individual's genetic information, doctors can make more accurate diagnoses, predict disease risks, and prescribe personalized treatment plans.

Genomic research plays a pivotal role in personalized medicine. The Human Genome Project, completed in 2003, was a significant milestone in genomic research, as it sequenced and mapped the human genome. Since then, there have been remarkable advancements in sequencing technologies, enabling faster and more cost-effective sequencing of individual genomes. In Germany, the field of genomics has seen substantial growth, with several research institutions and companies actively contributing to genomic research.

The application of personalized medicine in Germany has the potential to revolutionize healthcare. By identifying genetic markers associated with diseases, doctors can detect diseases at an early stage when they are most treatable. This approach can lead to more effective treatments and improved patient outcomes. Moreover, personalized medicine can help avoid unnecessary treatments, reducing healthcare costs and minimizing adverse side effects.

Germany has been at the forefront of personalized medicine, with leading academic institutions and hospitals embracing this approach. The country has established dedicated research centers and collaborations to drive genomic research and translate it into clinical practice. Additionally, Germany has implemented policies and regulations to ensure the ethical use of genomic data and protect patient privacy.

While personalized medicine holds great promise, challenges exist in its widespread implementation. One major challenge is the integration of genomic data into routine clinical practice. Healthcare professionals need to be trained in genomic medicine, and infrastructure must be established to handle the vast amount of genomic data generated.

In conclusion, personalized medicine and genomic research have the potential to transform the medical scope in Germany. The precise understanding of an individual's genetic makeup opens new avenues for disease prevention, diagnosis, and treatment. However, the successful integration of personalized medicine into routine healthcare requires ongoing research, investments, and collaborations to ensure its benefits reach all patients. By embracing personalized medicine, Germany can position itself as a global leader in providing innovative and patient-centric healthcare solutions.

Telemedicine and Remote Patient Monitoring

In recent years, the field of medicine has witnessed a revolutionary transformation with the advent of telemedicine and remote patient monitoring technologies. These innovative solutions have the potential to significantly impact the medical scope in Germany, improving patient care, increasing accessibility, and reducing healthcare costs.

Telemedicine refers to the use of telecommunications technology to provide medical services remotely. It allows healthcare professionals to diagnose, treat, and monitor patients without the need for in-person visits. This is particularly beneficial for patients living in rural or remote areas, where access to specialized healthcare services may be limited. Telemedicine enables these individuals to receive quality care from the comfort of their own homes.

Remote patient monitoring takes telemedicine a step further by utilizing wearable devices and sensors to collect and transmit patient data in real-time. These devices can monitor vital signs, such as heart rate, blood pressure, and glucose levels, allowing healthcare providers to track patients' health conditions continuously. This data can be analyzed to detect any anomalies or changes, enabling early intervention and preventive measures.

One of the significant advantages of telemedicine and remote patient monitoring is the improved convenience and accessibility for patients. Through video consultations and virtual visits, patients can avoid long travel times and waiting rooms, leading to more efficient care. This is particularly relevant in Germany, where the aging population and the increasing prevalence of chronic diseases require a more patient-centered approach to healthcare.

Additionally, telemedicine and remote patient monitoring have the potential to reduce healthcare costs significantly. By enabling early detection and intervention, these technologies can help prevent complications and hospital readmissions, ultimately saving resources. Moreover, they can reduce the burden on the healthcare system by managing non-emergency cases remotely, freeing up hospital beds and healthcare professionals for more critical cases.

However, while telemedicine and remote patient monitoring have shown great promise, there are still challenges to overcome. Ensuring data privacy and security, integrating these technologies into existing healthcare systems, and addressing reimbursement models are some of the hurdles that need to be addressed.

In conclusion, telemedicine and remote patient monitoring hold immense potential in transforming the medical scope in Germany. They offer improved accessibility, convenience, and cost-effectiveness, ultimately leading to better patient outcomes. As technology continues to advance, it is crucial for healthcare stakeholders to embrace these innovations and work towards their widespread implementation to shape the future of medicine in Germany.

Integrative Medicine and Complementary Therapies

Integrative medicine and complementary therapies have gained significant attention in recent years as alternative approaches to traditional medicine. In Germany, these practices have become an integral part of the medical scope, offering patients a holistic and comprehensive approach to healthcare. In this subchapter, we will explore the concept of integrative medicine and the various complementary therapies available in Germany.

Integrative medicine focuses on treating the whole person, taking into account their physical, emotional, and mental well-being. It combines conventional medical practices with evidence-based complementary therapies to provide patients with a personalized treatment plan. This approach recognizes that optimal health is achieved through the integration of different medical systems and practices, ultimately leading to better patient outcomes.

Germany has been at the forefront of integrative medicine, with numerous clinics and hospitals offering a wide range of complementary therapies. These therapies include acupuncture, herbal medicine, homeopathy, naturopathy, and mind-body techniques such as meditation and yoga. Patients have the option to choose from a diverse array of treatments, tailored to their unique needs and preferences.

One of the key advantages of integrative medicine is its focus on prevention and wellness. Complementary therapies, such as acupuncture and herbal medicine, have been shown to be effective in managing chronic conditions, reducing pain, and improving overall well-being. By incorporating these therapies into their treatment plans, patients have reported reduced reliance on pharmaceutical medications and improved quality of life.

In Germany, integrative medicine is supported by a strong regulatory framework. The German Medical Association has recognized certain complementary therapies as legitimate medical practices, ensuring that qualified practitioners adhere to strict standards and guidelines. This regulation provides patients with the assurance that they are receiving safe and effective treatments.

Moreover, the German healthcare system has recognized the value of integrative medicine by including certain complementary therapies in health insurance coverage. This has made these treatments more accessible and affordable for patients, encouraging them to explore these options as part of their healthcare journey.

In conclusion, integrative medicine and complementary therapies have revolutionized the medical scope in Germany. They offer patients a holistic and personalized approach to healthcare, focusing on prevention and overall well-being. With a diverse range of therapies available, patients can choose the treatments that align with their values and preferences. The strong regulatory framework and inclusion in health insurance coverage further solidify the importance of these practices in the future of medicine in Germany.

Rehabilitation and Physical Therapy Innovations

In recent years, Germany has emerged as a global leader in medical advancements, particularly in the field of rehabilitation and physical therapy. As the demand for specialized healthcare services continues to rise, the country has been at the forefront of developing innovative approaches and technologies to improve patient outcomes and quality of life. This subchapter explores some of the groundbreaking rehabilitation and physical therapy innovations that are shaping the future of medicine in Germany.

One of the most significant advancements in this field is the integration of robotic technology into rehabilitation programs. Robotic exoskeletons and devices have revolutionized the way patients recover from debilitating injuries or illnesses. These state-of-the-art machines assist patients in regaining strength and mobility by providing support and guidance during therapy sessions. With the help of sensors and artificial intelligence, these devices can adapt to individual needs and track progress over time, ensuring personalized and effective treatment.

Germany is also leading the way in the development of virtual reality (VR) and augmented reality (AR) technologies for rehabilitation purposes. By creating immersive and interactive environments, these technologies offer patients a unique and engaging experience that enhances their rehabilitation process. VR and AR can be used to simulate real-life scenarios, such as walking on uneven terrain or performing specific tasks, allowing patients to practice and improve their motor skills in a safe and controlled environment.

Furthermore, Germany is investing heavily in telemedicine and remote rehabilitation solutions, which have become even more crucial during the COVID-19 pandemic. Through video consultations and remote monitoring, patients can receive expert guidance and support from the comfort of their homes, reducing the need for physical visits to healthcare facilities. This approach not only improves access to care, particularly for those in rural or underserved areas, but also enables healthcare professionals to track patients' progress more closely and adjust their treatment plans accordingly.

In conclusion, Germany's commitment to innovation and excellence in the field of rehabilitation and physical therapy is transforming the way patients recover and regain their independence. Through the integration of robotic technology, virtual and augmented reality, and telemedicine solutions, the country is revolutionizing the rehabilitation process and improving patient outcomes. These advancements not only benefit patients directly but also contribute to the overall efficiency and effectiveness of the medical scope in Germany. With continued investment and research in this area, Germany is poised to remain a global leader in rehabilitation and physical therapy innovations for years to come.

Chapter 6: Enhancing Healthcare Delivery and Access

Efficient Hospital Management Systems

In the ever-evolving landscape of healthcare, the need for efficient hospital management systems has become paramount. As medical practices and technologies advance, it has become crucial for hospitals to streamline their operations and enhance patient care. This subchapter explores the various aspects of efficient hospital management systems and their significance in the medical scope of Germany.

Hospital management systems encompass a wide range of processes and technologies that enable hospitals to run smoothly and effectively. From patient registration to discharge, these systems ensure seamless coordination and communication among various departments, healthcare professionals, and support staff. By integrating electronic health records (EHRs), appointment scheduling, billing, and inventory management, hospitals can optimize their operations, reduce administrative burdens, and focus more on patient care.

In Germany, where the medical scope is renowned for its high standards and efficiency, hospital management systems play a vital role in maintaining the country's healthcare excellence. These systems allow hospitals to efficiently manage patient data, track medical histories, and facilitate communication among healthcare providers. By digitizing medical records, hospitals can reduce errors and improve overall patient safety. Furthermore, efficient hospital management systems enable better resource allocation, ensuring that medical supplies, equipment, and personnel are utilized optimally.

One of the key benefits of implementing efficient hospital management systems is the ability to enhance patient experience. With streamlined processes, patients can experience reduced waiting times, improved access to healthcare services, and better communication with their healthcare providers. These systems also empower patients to access their medical records, test results, and appointments online, offering convenience and fostering patient engagement.

Moreover, efficient hospital management systems contribute to cost savings and resource optimization. By automating various administrative tasks, hospitals can significantly reduce paperwork and eliminate unnecessary expenses. Efficient inventory management systems minimize stockouts and overstocking, leading to cost-effective procurement practices. Additionally, these systems can provide valuable insights through data analytics, allowing hospitals to identify areas for improvement and make informed decisions regarding resource allocation and budget planning.

In conclusion, efficient hospital management systems are indispensable in the medical scope of Germany. By leveraging technology and streamlining processes, hospitals can enhance patient care, improve resource allocation, and optimize operations. As the future of medicine advances, the adoption of efficient hospital management systems will continue to play a crucial role in maintaining Germany's position as a leader in healthcare innovation and excellence.

E-Health Records and Health Information Exchange

Health Insurance Reforms and Universal Coverage

In recent years, health insurance reforms and the pursuit of universal coverage have become hot topics within the medical scope in Germany. As the healthcare landscape continues to evolve, it is essential for all individuals to understand the reforms being implemented and their impact on the German healthcare system.

Germany has long been renowned for its robust healthcare system, which is based on a dual public-private model. Traditionally, individuals have had the choice between statutory health insurance (SHI) and private health insurance (PHI). However, with the aim of achieving universal coverage and ensuring equal access to healthcare for all citizens, recent reforms have sought to address the gaps and challenges within the existing system.

One of the key reforms is the strengthening of the SHI system. Statutory health insurance covers the majority of the German population and is financed through contributions from employees and employers. The recent reforms have focused on improving the financial stability and sustainability of SHI, ensuring that it can continue to provide comprehensive coverage to its members. This includes measures such as adjusting contribution rates, implementing cost containment strategies, and promoting transparency in healthcare pricing.

Another significant reform is the expansion of coverage for previously underserved populations. Germany has taken steps to ensure that vulnerable groups, such as the self-employed and low-income individuals, have access to affordable health insurance. This has been achieved through the introduction of a mandatory health insurance scheme for previously uninsured individuals, thus moving closer to achieving universal coverage.

Furthermore, reforms have also aimed to enhance the quality and efficiency of healthcare delivery. This includes the promotion of digital health solutions, such as electronic health records and telemedicine, to improve access to care, reduce administrative burdens, and enhance patient outcomes. Additionally, there has been a renewed focus on preventive care and health promotion, with the recognition that investing in preventive measures can lead to significant long-term cost savings.

Overall, the ongoing health insurance reforms in Germany are driven by the goal of achieving universal coverage and ensuring that all citizens have access to high-quality healthcare. These reforms not only work towards eliminating disparities within the healthcare system but also aim to create a more sustainable and efficient model for the future. By understanding these reforms and their implications, individuals can actively engage in the healthcare system and contribute to the improvement of medical care in Germany.

Improving Rural and Remote Healthcare Services

As Germany continues to make significant strides in the field of medicine, it is crucial to address the challenges faced by rural and remote areas when it comes to accessing healthcare services. The Future of Medicine in Germany: Innovations and Trends aims to shed light on the initiatives and innovations that are being implemented to bridge this gap and ensure that all citizens have equal access to quality healthcare.

Rural and remote areas in Germany often face unique healthcare challenges due to their geographical location and limited resources. One of the key issues is the shortage of healthcare professionals in these areas, making it difficult for residents to receive timely medical attention. To address this, innovative solutions such as telemedicine and mobile healthcare units have been introduced.

Telemedicine, which involves using digital communication technology to provide remote healthcare services, has emerged as a game-changer in rural areas. By leveraging video consultations and remote monitoring, patients can now receive medical advice and prescriptions without the need for physical visits to hospitals or clinics. This not only saves time and money but also ensures that medical expertise is accessible to all, regardless of their location.

Furthermore, mobile healthcare units have proven to be effective in reaching remote communities. These units are equipped with essential medical equipment and staffed by healthcare professionals who travel to underserved areas, providing preventive care, screenings, and basic treatments. This initiative has proven to be invaluable in diagnosing conditions at an early stage and preventing them from worsening due to lack of access to healthcare.

In addition to these technological advancements, the German government has also taken steps to incentivize healthcare professionals to work in rural areas. Through initiatives such as loan forgiveness programs and financial incentives, medical practitioners are encouraged to establish their practices in underserved regions. This not only ensures that rural areas have access to medical professionals but also helps in retaining local talent.

Improving rural and remote healthcare services is not only a matter of equal access but also contributes to the overall health and well-being of the entire nation. By addressing the challenges faced by these areas and implementing innovative solutions, Germany is moving towards a future where healthcare is accessible to all, regardless of their geographical location.

The Future of Medicine in Germany: Innovations and Trends aims to inspire readers to understand the importance of improving rural and remote healthcare services and the role they can play in supporting these initiatives. By highlighting the progress made and the potential for further advancements, this subchapter seeks to empower professionals within the medical scope in Germany and engage them in finding innovative solutions to bridge the healthcare gap for rural and remote communities.

Chapter 7: Ethical and Legal Implications in Medicine

Patient Privacy and Data Protection

In an era where technology is rapidly transforming the medical field, patient privacy and data protection have become critical issues in Germany's medical scope. As advancements in healthcare technologies and data analytics continue to revolutionize patient care, it is essential to address the challenges and opportunities associated with patient privacy and data protection.

The protection of patient privacy is a fundamental principle in the German healthcare system. It is enshrined in various laws and regulations, such as the General Data Protection Regulation (GDPR) and the Federal Data Protection Act (BDSG). These laws aim to safeguard patients' personal and sensitive information, ensuring that it is collected, processed, and stored in a secure and ethical manner.

One of the primary concerns in patient privacy is the collection and use of health data. With the advent of electronic health records (EHRs) and wearable devices, vast amounts of personal health information are being generated and shared. While these advancements offer immense potential for personalized medicine and improved patient outcomes, they also pose privacy risks. Therefore, strict protocols and encryption techniques must be implemented to protect patient data from unauthorized access and breaches.

To ensure patient privacy, healthcare providers in Germany are required to obtain informed consent from patients before collecting their data. Patients have the right to know how their data will be used and shared, giving them control over their personal information. Additionally, healthcare professionals must adhere to strict protocols when sharing patient data with third parties, ensuring that it is done securely and only for legitimate purposes.

Data protection goes hand in hand with patient privacy. It involves establishing robust security measures to prevent unauthorized access, data breaches, and cyber-attacks. Healthcare organizations must invest in state-of-the-art cybersecurity systems, regularly update their software, and train their staff on data protection protocols. Additionally, anonymization and pseudonymization techniques can be utilized to minimize the risk of re-identification of patients from their health data.

While patient privacy and data protection present challenges, they also offer opportunities for innovation and collaboration. Advancements in blockchain technology, for instance, hold promise in ensuring secure and transparent sharing of patient data across different healthcare providers. Collaborative efforts between researchers, policymakers, and technology experts are essential to develop robust frameworks that protect patient privacy while allowing for meaningful data analysis and research.

In conclusion, patient privacy and data protection are crucial aspects of Germany's medical scope. Striking a balance between leveraging technology for improved patient care and safeguarding patient privacy is vital. Through robust laws, regulations, and collaborative efforts, Germany can continue to lead the way in ensuring patient privacy and data protection in the future of medicine.

Ethical Considerations in Medical Research

In recent years, medical research has made significant advancements, leading to the development of innovative treatments and therapies. However, these advancements have also raised several ethical considerations that require careful examination. This subchapter aims to shed light on the ethical considerations in medical research, particularly focusing on the medical scope in Germany.

One of the primary ethical concerns in medical research is the protection of human participants. Researchers have a responsibility to ensure the well-being and safety of individuals involved in their studies. In Germany, stringent regulations and guidelines are in place to safeguard the rights and welfare of research participants. These include obtaining informed consent, ensuring privacy and confidentiality, and minimizing potential harm.

Another important consideration is the equitable distribution of the benefits and burdens of medical research. Germany, as a leading country in medical innovation, must ensure that research benefits are accessible to all segments of society. It is crucial to address any potential biases or disparities, such as gender, age, socioeconomic status, or geographic location, to ensure equal access to healthcare advancements.

Transparency and integrity are vital ethical principles in medical research. Researchers must disclose any conflicts of interest or funding sources that may influence their work. In Germany, funding bodies and research institutions have established rigorous protocols to maintain transparency and integrity throughout the research process. Open access to research findings and data sharing also contribute to the advancement of scientific knowledge and promote accountability.

The use of animals in medical research is another ethical aspect that requires careful consideration. While animal studies play a crucial role in understanding diseases and developing treatments, it is essential to minimize animal suffering and ensure the ethical treatment of research animals. Germany has implemented strict regulations for animal research, enforcing the principles of the 3Rs: replacement, reduction, and refinement.

Lastly, the ethical considerations in medical research extend to the dissemination of research findings. It is crucial for researchers to communicate their results accurately, avoiding any exaggeration or misrepresentation. This ensures the integrity of scientific knowledge and prevents potential harm to patients or the public.

In conclusion, ethical considerations play a vital role in medical research in Germany. The protection of human participants, equitable distribution of benefits, transparency, and integrity, animal welfare, and accurate dissemination of findings are key areas that demand attention. By upholding these ethical principles, Germany can continue to foster medical innovation while ensuring the well-being and trust of its citizens.

Legal Framework for Medical Innovations

Introduction:

In recent years, medical innovations have revolutionized the healthcare sector, improving patient outcomes and transforming the way healthcare is delivered. In Germany, a country known for its advancements in medical research and technology, the legal framework plays a crucial role in promoting and regulating medical innovations. This subchapter aims to provide an overview of the legal framework for medical innovations in Germany, catering to a broad audience interested in the medical scope in Germany.

1. Regulatory Authorities:
Germany has a well-established regulatory framework for medical innovations, ensuring that new technologies and treatments meet stringent safety and efficacy standards. The Federal Institute for Drugs and Medical Devices (BfArM) and the Paul Ehrlich Institute (PEI) are two key regulatory authorities responsible for granting marketing authorizations and overseeing clinical trials for pharmaceuticals and medical devices.

2. Clinical Trials:
Clinical trials are an essential part of the medical innovation process. In Germany, clinical trials are subject to rigorous ethical and legal requirements, ensuring patient safety and data protection. The subchapter will highlight the key regulations governing clinical trials, such as the Medicines Act and the Medical Devices Act, and provide an overview of the approval process.

3. Intellectual Property Rights:
Protecting intellectual property is crucial for incentivizing medical innovation. Germany has a robust system for granting patents and

copyrights, ensuring that innovators can reap the benefits of their discoveries. The subchapter will explore the various forms of intellectual property protection available in Germany and discuss their significance in the medical field.

4.   Data   Protection   and   Privacy: Medical innovations often rely on the collection and analysis of large amounts of patient data. Germany has stringent data protection laws, such as the General Data Protection Regulation (GDPR), which safeguard patient privacy and ensure the secure handling of sensitive medical information. The subchapter will delve into the legal requirements for data protection in medical research and innovation.

5.   Reimbursement   and   Market   Access: For medical innovations to reach patients, they must be adequately reimbursed and granted market access. Germany has a complex reimbursement system governed by the Federal Joint Committee (G-BA), which evaluates the added benefit of new treatments. The subchapter will outline the reimbursement process and discuss the challenges innovators face in gaining market access.

Conclusion:
The legal framework for medical innovations in Germany plays a pivotal role in fostering advancements in the medical field. By ensuring patient safety, protecting intellectual property, and promoting market access, these regulations contribute to the overall growth and success of the medical scope in Germany. Understanding the legal framework is crucial for all stakeholders involved in medical innovations, as it helps navigate the complex regulatory landscape and paves the way for the future of medicine in Germany.

Medical Malpractice and Liability

In the ever-evolving field of medicine, where advancements in technology and innovative treatments are constantly emerging, the issue of medical malpractice and liability remains a critical concern. This subchapter aims to shed light on the intricacies of medical malpractice in Germany, while also addressing the broader scope of the medical field in the country.

Medical malpractice refers to the negligence or wrongful actions of healthcare professionals that result in harm or injury to a patient. While the majority of medical practitioners in Germany provide exceptional care and adhere to the highest standards, instances of medical malpractice can still occur. It is crucial to understand the legal framework in place to protect patients and ensure accountability for medical professionals.

Germany has a comprehensive legal system that governs medical malpractice cases. The civil law code, known as the Bürgerliches Gesetzbuch (BGB), provides the foundation for medical liability claims. Patients who believe they have been a victim of medical malpractice can seek compensation through civil litigation. However, proving medical malpractice can be challenging, requiring expert opinions and evidence to demonstrate a breach of the duty of care.

To address the complexities of medical malpractice, Germany has established medical liability insurance. Healthcare providers are required to carry professional indemnity insurance, ensuring that patients receive compensation for damages resulting from medical negligence. This system not only safeguards patients but also protects healthcare professionals from financial ruin in the event of a malpractice claim.

In the broader context of the medical field in Germany, it is essential to recognize the significant advancements and trends shaping the industry. Germany boasts a robust healthcare system known for its cutting-edge research, state-of-the-art medical facilities, and highly skilled healthcare professionals. From pioneering treatments in areas such as oncology and neurology to embracing digital health technologies, Germany continues to be at the forefront of medical innovation.

Moreover, the German medical scope encompasses various disciplines, including primary care, specialized medicine, and alternative therapies. The country's emphasis on preventive care and patient-centered approaches has contributed to its reputation for delivering high-quality healthcare.

Understanding medical malpractice and liability is vital for all individuals, including patients, healthcare professionals, and policymakers. By recognizing the legal framework and the broader medical landscape in Germany, stakeholders can work together to ensure patient safety, foster innovation, and uphold the highest standards of medical care.

In conclusion, this subchapter highlights the importance of addressing medical malpractice and liability in Germany. It explores the legal framework in place to protect patients and hold healthcare professionals accountable. Additionally, it provides an overview of the medical scope in Germany, emphasizing the country's commitment to innovation and patient-centered care. By examining these aspects, this subchapter aims to promote a comprehensive understanding of the future of medicine in Germany.

Chapter 8: Future Challenges and Opportunities

Aging Population and Geriatric Healthcare

As the world continues to evolve, the population in Germany is experiencing a significant shift towards an aging society. This demographic change brings about various challenges and opportunities, especially within the scope of medical care. In this subchapter, we will explore the implications of the aging population on geriatric healthcare in Germany and discuss the innovative trends that are shaping the future of medicine in this field.

Germany, like many developed countries, is witnessing a remarkable increase in life expectancy. While this is undoubtedly a positive outcome of advancements in healthcare, it also poses unique challenges. The aging population requires specialized medical attention that caters to their unique needs and conditions. This necessitates a reevaluation of the healthcare system to ensure that it can provide comprehensive and quality care to older adults.

Geriatric healthcare in Germany is multidimensional, encompassing various aspects such as preventive care, chronic disease management, rehabilitation, and palliative care. With a growing number of older adults, there is an increasing demand for specialized healthcare professionals who can address the specific needs of this segment of the population. This demand has led to the emergence of innovative medical training programs and the development of specialized geriatric care centers across the country.

One crucial aspect of geriatric healthcare in Germany is the promotion of healthy aging and preventive measures. Recognizing the importance of proactive healthcare, the government and healthcare providers have been investing in programs that focus on promoting healthy lifestyles, disease prevention, and early detection. These initiatives aim to reduce the burden on the healthcare system by preventing or delaying the onset of age-related diseases.

Furthermore, advancements in technology and digital healthcare solutions are revolutionizing the field of geriatric medicine. Telemedicine, remote patient monitoring, and wearable devices are increasingly being utilized to provide personalized care and monitor the health status of older adults. These technologies not only enhance patient autonomy but also enable healthcare providers to deliver timely interventions and improve overall healthcare outcomes.

In conclusion, the aging population in Germany is driving significant changes in the healthcare landscape, particularly within the field of geriatric medicine. The increasing demand for specialized care and the need for preventive measures are reshaping the medical scope in Germany. By investing in innovative training programs, specialized care centers, and digital healthcare solutions, Germany is at the forefront of addressing the unique challenges posed by an aging population. Embracing these trends and innovations will ensure that the future of geriatric healthcare in Germany is patient-centered, efficient, and sustainable.

Mental Health and Psychiatric Care

In recent years, mental health has gained significant attention worldwide, and Germany is no exception. The importance of mental well-being and the need for quality psychiatric care have become increasingly apparent. This subchapter aims to shed light on the current state of mental health and psychiatric care in Germany, focusing on the innovations and trends that are shaping the future of medicine in this field.

Germany has long been recognized for its advanced medical care, and mental health is no different. The country boasts a comprehensive healthcare system, which includes a well-established network of mental health services. With a growing awareness of mental health issues, Germany's medical scope has expanded to address the increasing demand for psychiatric care.

One of the key innovations in mental health care in Germany is the integration of mental health services into primary care. This approach recognizes the interconnection between physical and mental health and aims to provide comprehensive care to patients. By incorporating mental health professionals into primary care settings, individuals can receive timely and holistic treatment, reducing the stigma associated with seeking help for mental health issues.

Additionally, Germany has witnessed a surge in technological advancements that are revolutionizing psychiatric care. Telemedicine, for instance, has gained popularity, allowing individuals to access mental health services remotely. This technology is particularly beneficial for those in rural areas with limited access to healthcare facilities. Virtual therapy sessions and online support groups provide convenience and anonymity, fostering a more accessible and inclusive mental health system.

Furthermore, Germany is investing in the training and education of mental health professionals to meet the growing demand for their services. Specialized programs and certifications are being developed to ensure that healthcare providers have the necessary skills and knowledge to deliver high-quality mental health care. This commitment to professional development is crucial in ensuring that individuals receive evidence-based and compassionate care.

In conclusion, mental health and psychiatric care are integral components of the medical scope in Germany. With a focus on integration, technology, and professional development, the country is working towards a future where mental health is treated with the same importance as physical health. By staying at the forefront of medical innovation and trends, Germany is poised to provide comprehensive mental health care to all its citizens, ensuring a healthier and happier population.

Integrating Traditional and Modern Medicine

In today's rapidly evolving medical landscape, the integration of traditional and modern medicine has emerged as a topic of great importance. This subchapter explores the synergies and potential benefits of combining traditional and modern medical practices in Germany, shedding light on the current trends and innovations that are shaping the future of medicine in the country.

Germany has a rich history of traditional medicine, with practices such as herbal medicine, acupuncture, and homeopathy deeply rooted in its cultural heritage. These traditional practices have been passed down through generations and have continued to gain popularity among patients seeking alternative treatments. However, the rise of modern medicine and its evidence-based approach has also played a significant role in shaping the medical landscape in Germany.

The integration of traditional and modern medicine offers a holistic approach to healthcare, addressing the physical, emotional, and spiritual well-being of patients. It recognizes the value of both approaches and seeks to leverage the strengths of each to optimize patient outcomes. By combining the centuries-old wisdom of traditional medicine with the advances in modern medical technology, practitioners can offer a comprehensive range of treatment options.

One of the key trends in the integration of traditional and modern medicine in Germany is the collaboration between practitioners from different disciplines. This interdisciplinary approach allows for the exchange of knowledge and expertise, enabling practitioners to develop innovative treatment protocols that draw on the best of both worlds. For instance, a cancer patient may receive chemotherapy treatment alongside acupuncture therapy to manage side effects and improve overall well-being.

Another notable trend is the increasing acceptance and recognition of traditional medicine within the German healthcare system. In recent years, traditional practices such as acupuncture and homeopathy have been included in health insurance coverage, allowing more patients to access these treatments. This integration has also led to the establishment of specialized clinics and centers that offer integrative medicine, providing a platform for collaboration between traditional and modern medicine practitioners.

However, the integration of traditional and modern medicine is not without its challenges. One of the key obstacles is the need for standardized regulations and guidelines to ensure the safety and efficacy of traditional practices. As traditional medicine often relies on individualized treatments and subjective assessment, there is a need for robust research and evidence-based studies to validate its effectiveness.

In conclusion, the integration of traditional and modern medicine in Germany offers a promising path for the future of healthcare. By combining the strengths of both approaches, practitioners can provide a more comprehensive and patient-centered care. This integration not only expands treatment options but also fosters collaboration, innovation, and ultimately, improved patient outcomes. As the healthcare landscape continues to evolve, the integration of traditional and modern medicine will undoubtedly play a vital role in shaping the medical scope in Germany.

Global Collaboration and Medical Diplomacy

In today's interconnected world, global collaboration and medical diplomacy play a pivotal role in shaping the future of medicine in Germany. As a country known for its cutting-edge advancements in healthcare, Germany has recognized the importance of fostering international partnerships to drive innovation, exchange knowledge, and improve healthcare outcomes not only within its borders but also globally.

The scope of medical practice in Germany extends beyond its own healthcare system, as the country actively engages in collaborations with international organizations, research institutions, and medical professionals worldwide. This subchapter explores the significance of global collaboration in the context of medical diplomacy and its impact on the future of medicine in Germany.

One of the key benefits of global collaboration is the exchange of medical expertise and best practices. By collaborating with experts from different countries, Germany gains access to a diverse range of medical knowledge, enabling the country to stay at the forefront of medical research and innovation. This knowledge exchange also benefits German medical professionals, who can learn from their international counterparts and incorporate novel approaches into their own practices.

Medical diplomacy, on the other hand, focuses on using healthcare initiatives as a means of fostering diplomatic relationships and promoting peace. Germany's commitment to medical diplomacy is evident through its participation in international health organizations such as the World Health Organization (WHO), where it actively contributes to global health policies and initiatives. Through medical diplomacy, Germany not only showcases its expertise but also establishes itself as a trusted partner in addressing global health challenges.

Moreover, global collaboration and medical diplomacy have a direct impact on the medical scope in Germany. By engaging in international partnerships, Germany attracts foreign medical professionals, researchers, and students who contribute to the diversity and knowledge enrichment of its healthcare system. This influx of talent enhances the overall medical expertise available in the country, leading to improved patient care and outcomes.

Furthermore, global collaboration allows Germany to contribute to medical research and development on a global scale. By participating in international clinical trials, sharing data, and collaborating on research projects, Germany plays a significant role in advancing medical knowledge and developing innovative treatments that benefit patients worldwide.

In conclusion, global collaboration and medical diplomacy are instrumental in shaping the future of medicine in Germany. Through partnerships and diplomatic initiatives, Germany gains access to international expertise, fosters innovation, and establishes itself as a global leader in healthcare. As the country continues to embrace global collaboration, the medical scope in Germany will further expand, benefiting both its citizens and the global community at large.

Chapter 9: Conclusion

Summary of Findings

In this subchapter, we aim to provide a comprehensive summary of the key findings and trends discussed throughout the book "The Future of Medicine in Germany: Innovations and Trends." This summary is intended for a diverse audience, including individuals interested in the medical scope in Germany.

1.   Healthcare   System   Overview: We begin by giving an overview of the German healthcare system, which is known for its universal coverage and high-quality care. The system is characterized by a strong emphasis on preventive medicine, patient-centered care, and a well-developed infrastructure.

2.   Technological   Innovations: One of the major findings in this book is the significant role played by technological innovations in shaping the future of medicine in Germany. We explore how artificial intelligence, telemedicine, and digital health solutions are revolutionizing healthcare delivery, improving diagnostics, and enhancing patient outcomes.

3.   Precision   Medicine: The concept of precision medicine is gaining traction in Germany, and our research highlights how it is transforming the medical landscape. We delve into the advancements in genomics, personalized therapies, and biomarker identification, which are paving the way for more targeted and effective treatments.

4. Integration of Traditional and Alternative Medicines: Germany has a rich history of integrating traditional and alternative medicines into its healthcare system. Our findings shed light on the

increasing acceptance of complementary therapies, such as acupuncture and herbal medicine, and how they are being integrated with conventional medicine to provide holistic patient care.

5.   Healthcare   Workforce:
We examine the challenges and opportunities surrounding the healthcare workforce in Germany. Our research highlights the need for a well-trained, diverse, and culturally competent workforce to meet the growing demands of an aging population and the influx of refugees.

6.   Future   Trends:
The book concludes with an analysis of future trends that will shape the medical landscape in Germany. We discuss the importance of data-driven healthcare, the rise of preventive medicine, and the increasing focus on patient empowerment through health literacy and shared decision-making.

Throughout this subchapter, we have presented a concise summary of the key findings and trends discussed in "The Future of Medicine in Germany: Innovations and Trends." Whether you are a medical professional, a policymaker, or simply interested in the medical scope in Germany, this summary provides valuable insights into the future of medicine and healthcare in the country.

Implications for the Future of Medicine in Germany

Germany has long been recognized as a global leader in the field of medicine, with a rich history of scientific breakthroughs and cutting-edge research. As we look ahead to the future, it is clear that the implications for the future of medicine in Germany are vast and promising. In this subchapter, we will explore some of the key trends and innovations that are shaping the medical scope in Germany and discuss the potential implications they hold for patients, healthcare professionals, and the overall healthcare system.

One of the most significant implications for the future of medicine in Germany is the integration of digital technologies and artificial intelligence (AI) into healthcare practices. The use of electronic health records, telemedicine, and remote patient monitoring are becoming increasingly common, enabling more personalized and efficient care. AI algorithms are being developed to aid in diagnosis and treatment decisions, revolutionizing the way healthcare is delivered. However, with these advancements come ethical and privacy concerns that need to be addressed to ensure patient trust and safety.

Another implication for the future of medicine in Germany is the increasing focus on preventive and personalized medicine. With a growing understanding of genetic and environmental factors that contribute to disease, there is a shift towards tailoring treatments to individual patients. Genetic testing and precision medicine are gaining importance, enabling doctors to prescribe targeted therapies that have the potential to improve patient outcomes and reduce healthcare costs in the long run.

Furthermore, the future of medicine in Germany will see an increased interdisciplinary collaboration and team-based care. The complexity of healthcare requires the expertise of various professionals, including doctors, nurses, pharmacists, and allied health professionals. Integrated care models are being developed to ensure seamless coordination and communication among different providers, ultimately leading to better patient outcomes and experiences.

Lastly, the future of medicine in Germany will be characterized by a greater emphasis on health promotion and disease prevention. As the burden of chronic diseases continues to rise, there is a growing recognition of the importance of lifestyle interventions and community-based programs. Public health initiatives, such as smoking cessation campaigns and obesity prevention programs, are being implemented to tackle these challenges and improve the overall health of the population.

In conclusion, the future of medicine in Germany holds immense potential and numerous implications for patients, healthcare professionals, and the healthcare system as a whole. The integration of digital technologies, the focus on personalized medicine, interdisciplinary collaboration, and a greater emphasis on preventive care are some of the key trends and innovations that will shape the medical scope in Germany. By embracing these changes and addressing the associated challenges, Germany can continue to lead the way in advancing healthcare and improving patient outcomes.

Recommendations for Policy and Practice

In recent years, the medical landscape in Germany has witnessed significant transformations and innovations. As we look towards the future, it is crucial to identify key recommendations for policies and practices that will shape the medical scope in Germany.

1. Strengthening Healthcare Infrastructure: One of the primary recommendations is to focus on strengthening the healthcare infrastructure in Germany. This includes increasing the number of hospitals, clinics, and healthcare centers, especially in underserved regions. Additionally, investing in state-of-the-art medical equipment and technologies will enhance the quality of care provided.

2. Promoting Research and Development: Germany has always been at the forefront of medical research and development. To continue this trend, policymakers should prioritize funding for research institutions and encourage collaboration between academia and industry. This will facilitate the development of innovative medical technologies, drugs, and treatment methods.

3. Enhancing Digital Healthcare: The digital revolution has the potential to revolutionize healthcare delivery. Policymakers should invest in digital health infrastructure, such as electronic health records and telemedicine platforms. These advancements will improve access to healthcare services, enable remote consultations, and enhance patient outcomes.

4. Addressing Workforce Shortages: Germany, like many other countries, is facing a shortage of healthcare professionals. Encouraging more students to pursue medical careers, providing financial incentives for healthcare professionals in underserved areas, and

streamlining the recognition process for foreign-trained doctors are some strategies to address this issue. Additionally, investing in continuous medical education and training programs will ensure that healthcare professionals are equipped with the latest knowledge and skills.

5. Fostering Interdisciplinary Collaboration: The future of medicine lies in interdisciplinary collaboration. Policymakers should encourage collaboration between different medical specialties, as well as foster partnerships between healthcare professionals, researchers, and technology experts. This interdisciplinary approach will lead to more comprehensive and personalized patient care.

6. Prioritizing Preventive Medicine: Prevention is better than cure. Policymakers should prioritize preventive medicine by promoting healthy lifestyles, providing affordable access to preventive screenings, and implementing public health campaigns. This will not only reduce the burden on the healthcare system but also improve overall population health.

In conclusion, the future of medicine in Germany depends on effective policies and practices. By focusing on strengthening healthcare infrastructure, promoting research and development, enhancing digital healthcare, addressing workforce shortages, fostering interdisciplinary collaboration, and prioritizing preventive medicine, Germany can ensure a robust and innovative medical scope that meets the needs of its population.

Milton Keynes UK
Ingram Content Group UK Ltd.
UKHW020930231123
433129UK00016B/845